THE SCIENCE OF SLEEP

THE SCIENCE OF SLEEP

ELIAS HARTLEY

CONTENTS

1	Introduction to the Importance of Sleep	1
2	The Biology and Physiology of Sleep	5
3	Neuroscience of Sleep	9
4	Sleep Disorders and Their Impact	11
5	The Psychology of Sleep	15
6	Sleep and Mental Health	19
7	Sleep and Physical Health	21
8	Sleep Hygiene and Best Practices	25
9	Technology and Sleep	29
10	Sleep Across the Lifespan	31
11	Cultural and Societal Perspectives on Sleep	35
12	Sleep Research Methodologies	39
13	Future Trends in Sleep Science	43
14	Conclusion and Practical Tips for Better Sleep	47

Copyright © 2024 by Elias Hartley
All rights reserved. No part of this book may be reproduced in any manner whatsoever without written permission except in the case of brief quotations embodied in critical articles and reviews.
First Printing, 2024

CHAPTER 1

Introduction to the Importance of Sleep

This chapter is intended to increase your understanding of the role of sleep so that you can make the necessary changes to ensure that those sixty days spent lying in bed each year pass peacefully and productively. Schoolchildren aged five or six years old are recommended to sleep for twelve hours a night; this reduces to a mere eight or nine hours by the age of eighteen. If you are a healthy adult getting less than eight hours of sleep per night, then you are probably sleep deprived. Even six hours a night may not be enough.

Almost everyone will be familiar with many of the inconvenient side effects of a bad night's sleep: they are irritable, have little or no energy, the ability to concentrate falls away, and a range of aches and pains can also result. In the short run, one uncomfortable night can impact on people's performance markedly. Yet it's what sleep does for the body in the longer term that really matters. The average adult spends nearly a third of their lives asleep, which makes the time we spend lying down a surprisingly important issue. When you are lying there counting sheep, something extraordinarily serious is occurring; every minute that you are asleep, thousands of your body's chemicals are buzzing around regulating and healing different parts of your body. Many different processes are being regulated and instigated during sleep, and your body won't go on functioning smoothly if you habitually skimp on shuteye.

Defining Sleep

Is sleep rest? If not, what is it? It is almost impossible to observe sleep in another person or animal and know where the threshold separates the awake and asleep states. If sleep is not defined by posture or relaxation, by what is it defined? Finally, sleep is crucial to a healthy life, but its function is not known. What do you think sleep is? The appropriate definition of sleep is as difficult to decide as the definition of consciousness, about which there is extensive debate. Sleep may actually be easier to define than consciousness because there are more candidates for necessary and sufficient conditions.

Sleep is as important to living things as food and water. In fact, it is so important that we spend about one third of our lives doing it. Still, the function of sleep is not known, and there are many misconceptions about it. It is a surprising fact that scientists do not even know why we wake up from sleep.

Historical Perspectives on Sleep

Aristotle is recorded as writing that "a certain fish, I know not what, sleeps." In a similarly casual manner, the physician Galen, in the 2nd century AD, observed that all animals, as well as humans, are capable of sleeping. These ancient observations suggest that in the earliest recorded contemplation of sleep, the need for sleep is recognized, but that lack of sleep is not specifically cited as directly leading to death. In the early 20th century, once again people began to question what sleep's most critical functions actually were. Kleitman and Vogt commented that "there is no subject in the whole field of physiology where there is so little unanimity as in the explanation of the nature and purpose of sleep." In 1845, Marshall Hall suggested that the subjective sensation of fatigue prevented sudden continuous wakefulness. As soon as the fatigue had helped to produce the superficial diffusion of sensation that was associated with sleep onset, Hall suggested that the need to sleep, forcing the subject's involuntary nervous functions into the state necessary for sleep, could then take place. Since the realization that many of the effects of sleep are actually effects of sleep deprivation, sleep has been seen to be a restorative process that has a function of absolute importance. At the end of the 20th century, the idea that sleep is necessary to restore homeostatic imbalances that have developed during wakefulness was finally generally accepted, albeit without universal agreement on specifics.

We know sleep is important, but why do we sleep? Many people shrug this question off, thinking that it's just something we do. When we can't sleep, which is about half the time for most people at some point in their lives, we start to believe that sleep is critical for our bodies and minds to function normally because not sleeping definitely impacts both. Scientists and historians do agree that sleep is integral to living a healthy, functional life, and even though we can recognize the damage that comes from being sleep deprived, the exact reason that sleep is so necessary still isn't clear. Over time, there have been many different perspectives and theories regarding sleep, and scientists are coming to a consensus, considering research and scientific findings. Before delving into the modern science behind sleep, though, it's useful to consider some historical perspectives, especially for understanding the conclusions reached by modern scientists.

CHAPTER 2

The Biology and Physiology of Sleep

The brain does not simply shut down or go into a low-power state when we sleep. EEGs, electroencephalograms, of sleeping patients show different stages of electrical activity. There are two broad stages of sleep, non-rapid eye movement (NREM) sleep and rapid eye movement (REM) sleep. NREM sleep is also divided into three stages: N1, N2 and N3. While the electrical activities associated with the different stages are distinct, it is not completely clear what they represent. What is clear is that we need to go through this entire cycle of stages in order to experience the benefits of sleep, and by extension to avoid the hazards of sleep deprivation. This complete cycle usually takes about ninety minutes and is repeated four to five times during a night of sleep. Adults spend most of their time in N2 sleep. Blood pressure goes down during N3 sleep, although it is possible for it to go back up sporadically. Brain waves, eye movements, and the muscle twitches do not occur in N3 sleep, but the body is working hard. It is repairing muscles and tissue, stimulating growth and development, boosting the immune system, and building up energy for the next day.

Before going into tips to get better sleep, it is important to understand the function sleep serves. No one knows exactly why creatures need sleep, but we know that the ability to engage in extended periods of sleep would not have evolved if it were not essential. Sleep is fundamental to our brain and also is restorative to our body. It is our time to rest, recharge, and rejuvenate from a hard day's work. The different stages of sleep are another indicator that sleep is important. If the body really only needed an eight-hour rest, there would be no need to cycle through the various stages of sleep like a long play cycle. Those stages can also give us some clues as to what sleep functions may be. It might be something as simple as short circuits in the computation of a day's data.

Stages of Sleep

The stereotypical physiological pattern of REM sleep includes a decrease in respiratory rate and relative metabolic rate. Profound skeletal muscle atonia, altered thermoregulatory control, and, in the male, genital blood vasculature changes are also characteristic. REM sleep is also associated with an EEG characterized by low-voltage, high-frequency, and large amplitude waveforms. Collectively, these observations present a compelling picture of REM sleep as a distinctive brain state. Although REM sleep shares many of these features, physiological characteristics of NREM sleep are less salient than REM sleep, and state intensity can only be inferred through metabolic and neurophysiological variables. NREM sleep can be further characterized on the basis of EEG-coincident events, including spindles or K-complexes, and these more measured distinctions in state intensity may provide a better understanding of function.

During a normal night's sleep, the adult will cycle intermittently between NREM (non-rapid eye movement) sleep and REM sleep. The order of these sleep stages is NREM-REM-NREM-REM, and this cycle is often broken down further into multiple instances of shorter NREM-REM cycles. The length of the initial NREM sleep episodes is typically short, and the first REM episode occurs relatively soon after the onset of sleep. The REM episode that follows each NREM stage increases in duration for approximately the first 3/4 of the night and decreases in the last 1/4 of the night. However, the bulk of the discussion will focus on the structure and function of these two primary behavioral sleep states.

Circadian Rhythms

The biggest example of circadian rhythms can be seen with time zones. When you travel across time zones, your body has no idea that you did this. It is still on your time at home. It may take a while for you to adjust to the new time in your destination because of circadian rhythms. These circadian rhythms happen over a 24-hour time frame, usually regulated by the light and dark signals your brain receives. You need to sleep like 7-8 hours a night. Your body does this day in and day out like clockwork. This schedule is what works best for most people. What happens when you disrupt your sleep schedule? For most of us, nothing good comes from it. Routine is a settling force and it helps us get a good night's sleep.

Circadian rhythms are one of the most important factors when it comes to your daily success at work and at home. These rhythms act like small biological clocks that help control your sleep, wake, and activity periods. Have you ever noticed that right around the same time every day you start to feel drained and need a quick pick-me-up? It is because of your circadian rhythms. Your body does this based on how much time you have been awake, but also based on these little tiny biological clocks. You've heard the term internal body clock, right? Well, this is the team that is being referred to.

CHAPTER 3

Neuroscience of Sleep

The infographic has layers of comfort, tech innovations, and sleeping positions, but what's really going on during sleep? Sleep remains one of the most mysterious areas of neuroscience. Throughout evolution, sleep has never provided a direct benefit to survival, so we know that it is very important. Neuroscientists are currently exploring an enormous array of mechanisms to explain why sleep is important. It is generally agreed that sleep has both a recuperative and a firmly adaptive role. During sleep, the body can rest and repair itself, and the brain can arrange itself for the next set of waking tasks. Ironing out novel memories, repairing damaged neurons, and spreading the latest synaptic nutrients are all well-known functions of sleep. But why do we have to be unconscious while we do these things? Surely we are missing out on important evolutionary opportunities by not foraging, escaping from enemies, or seducing potential mates? It is a relatively simple question to ask, but considerably harder to answer.

Brain Regions and Sleep

One piece of evidence in favor of this theory is that many species sleep more after learning novel cues or performing difficult learning and memory tasks. Moving in the direction of effects induced by sleep deprivation, there is a large amount of research in favor of the theory that sleeping less negatively impacts performance in these tasks. Still another possibility is that one function of sleep is to maintain homeostasis. Different pieces of evidence support this theory.

Sleep is not random; it often appears quite structured. Given that people spend a full one-third of their lives asleep, it is reasonable to question why this is. Many theories have tried to address such a question, including the housekeeping theory. The variations between neuronal activity during wakefulness and sleep suggest that sleep can help the brain recover from the effects of activity during wakefulness. For example, during sleep, long-term synaptic strength is weakened in an activity-dependent manner, and CBF and interstitial space volume are increased. Additionally, during certain stages of sleep, there is evidence that neurons are finely tuned, which could help in improving performance or preparing the brain for learning future tasks. Other theories suggest that the most likely functions of sleep include learning and memory consolidation.

CHAPTER 4

Sleep Disorders and Their Impact

Regular exercise, not smoking, avoiding heavy meals, and maintaining an ideal weight can help to prevent primary insomnia or reduce its continuance. Numerous medications are available for insomnia, although it is important to balance benefits against potential adverse reactions, and second-line agents may be necessary after an initial trial of the first choice drug. Many new medications are being evaluated, and alternative treatments, such as herbal supplements or warm milk, are also being used to treat insomnia. Over-the-counter formulations are available, but when used long-term, they are associated with the highest rates of misuse and abuse, a particular problem in the elderly.

Sleep disorders include a number of conditions such as insomnia and restless legs syndrome. Twenty percent of healthy people between the ages of 20 and 50 have symptoms of inadequate sleep, and one-third of those people have one of two primary types of insomnia. These are either problems falling asleep or maintaining sleep, both of which cause significant impairment in social functioning the next day. Treatment options for these types of insomnia include both nonpharmacological and pharmacological interventions. Nonpharmacological approaches for acute insomnia include time-limited encouragement to allow sleep to happen, relaxation techniques, and education about sleep and how to improve it.

Insomnia

While it is the easiest thing in the world to ignore the signs that suggest we have insomnia, doing so has implications for health, mood, and mental agility. As we have seen, lack of adequate sleep can make people irritable, forgetful, and unable to concentrate or undertake tasks requiring significant memory or mental deployment. Insomnia also comes with worrisome consequences. People with chronic insomnia utilize more medical resources than others in their age group and are more likely to experience associated accidents. It has been estimated that driving while sleepy may be considered some four times more dangerous than driving while drunk. When we do admit we have a problem and seek advice, what solutions does sleep science offer? There are two broad approaches to improving the quality of our sleep, one of which addresses physical problems, while the other focuses on psychological or behavioral issues.

While most of us use the term "insomnia" to mean difficulty sleeping, it is a more profound concept than that. Insomnia occurs when a person can't get to sleep, can't stay asleep, and can't get back to sleep once awakened. It can persist for days, weeks, and sometimes years, and be caused by a variety of things. Insomnia can result from worry or stress, changes in the environment we normally sleep in, and alterations to our typical routines (work, etc.). It may also be due to medical problems, such as depression or other types of mental illness, obstructive sleep apnea, blocked breathing passages, excessive weight, or poorly controlled chronic illnesses. Medications can also cause insomnia, as well as consuming stimulants like caffeine or nicotine late in the day. Even alcohol can cause sleeplessness by altering the chemical makeup of sleep. Other examples are changes that occur during or after extended periods of international travel, when the body's internal clock is out of sync with the new time zone.

Sleep Apnea

There are two types of sleep apnea. Obstructive sleep apnea is caused by a blockage of the airway, usually when your soft palate collapses and tongue falls back. Central sleep apnea occurs when your brain fails to signal the muscles that control breathing. Combining both types is called complex sleep apnea syndrome. Sleep apnea is most commonly seen in men, those who are overweight, those who are over 40 years of age, have a family history of sleep apnea, get sinus infections, and have large tonsils, a large tongue, or a small jaw. Other contributing factors are injuries to the head and neck, allergies, sinus problems, smoking, and sedatives. Small children may also have sleep apnea, which can be caused by inflammation and enlarged tonsils.

Sleep apnea is characterized by pauses in breathing during sleep. People with severe cases can stop breathing hundreds of times during the night, from seconds to over a minute. In most cases, the person is unaware of these brief episodes. They wake up at the end of the night and feel tired throughout the day. This can lead to serious health problems due to chronic stress, a hallmark of sleep apnea. These health issues include frequent awakenings, low blood oxygen levels, poor sleep, heart disease, high blood pressure, heart failure, heart attack, stroke, diabetes, depression, headaches, decreased work productivity, and unsafe driving.

CHAPTER 5

The Psychology of Sleep

If dreaming does occur, it may exist as an independent state produced when sleep architecture is sufficiently modified by applying neurons and certain brainstem structures that function to make the complex and intricate criteria more complex and difficult. During the past several decades, interest in sleep-related phenomena and specific information about them have undergone a major transformation. Heats have been clarified regarding much of the story of sleep. Information is no longer so murky concerning how much sleep and what kind the different stages of sleep, when sleep takes place, and what are some of the things and processes operating in the sleeping brain and body. Is sleep enough to quote Milton? "Nature is fine in love, and often asleep," or is sleep "the brother to death"? Can sleep be considered merely an adaptive phase of behavior? Given the available evidence in favor of the adaptive component, an electrobiological basis is justified, but sleep should not be solely regarded as a biological necessity. Sleep also has a psychological or psychological capacity, and lack of sleep has far-reaching impact on our behaviors.

Sleep, believed to be a time of mental quietude, is not at all still and dormant as the popular imagery would have it. It is almost as busy at night as the body is during the day, as it is an important time for brain metabolism. Sleep has been the subject of great speculation and many theories. At the very core of many ongoing sleep controversies and the source of many lasting obstacles to understanding sleep is whether or not one consciously experiences activity that is going on when an individual is asleep. Many movements and actions going on during nocturnal sleep, such as leg jerking, disorganized repetitive thrashing or violence, mumbling, vocalizing, and angry-looking cursing, teeth grinding, nocturnal eating, connectedness jokes, music, and expressions of orgasm, are observed by an observer, but the sleeping individual is unaware of them.

Dreaming and REM Sleep

Since the beginning of recorded history, humans have been fascinated by dreams and their meaning. Dreams have led to predictions, to myths and legends, and to countless discussions of their interpretation. The ancient Greeks regarded the dream as a divine message. Until the Enlightenment, many believed that dreams were messages from the spirits inhabiting the dreamer's body. In 1953, experiments demonstrated a connection between dreaming and the stage of sleep known as rapid eye movement, or REM, sleep. During REM sleep, electroencephalographic records show that the brain is very active, the eyes move quickly and energy expenditure increases above the level of being awake but at rest. The electrical rhythms of the brain also change. Large, low-voltage, irregular brain waves replace the small, high-voltage, slow brain waves. Rapid eye movements are common. The heart beats irregularly, sometimes faster than 100 beats per minute, and blood pressure increases. These intense physiological activities are associated with reports of colored, vivid dreams.

Now we dream. We dream because we sleep, and only under such circumstances are our senses and imagination free. Often we are far away in dreamland; sometimes, however, in such close association with the actual sensations that the mind permits transference to sleep only as long as these are tolerable.

CHAPTER 6

Sleep and Mental Health

These findings reveal an incredibly important aspect of human sleep: it's a factor that operates at the very core of our existence, below the surface of whatever it is that constitutes "us." This suggests an almost unfathomably intimate connection between a person's sleep and themselves. What's more, sleep acts as a kind of gatekeeper to our mind; a filter placed across the bridge that connects body and brain. Once the function of this filter is disrupted, the way we function no longer flows smoothly. The way we feel and think dries out or twists and turns before connecting to where it ought to. The result is that at some level, our quality of life has been compromised due to the basic biological issue that is sleep. The evidence base on the importance of sleep for mental health may take a while to reach clinical practice, but meanwhile, we need to accept its implications. For anyone wishing to catch a glimpse of the proof, simply lift the lid of your own life after a poor night's sleep. Then pause to wonder what your brain would reveal if it could lift its own lid.

In the same way that sleep acts as a powerful bridge between body and mind, it also plays an important role in mental development and health. Over the past century, researchers have discovered that sleep benefits patients with a broad array of mental health problems including anxiety, depression, bipolar disorder, or schizophrenia, to name just a few. Correspondingly, insomnia—chronic, distorted, or inefficient sleep—can have a truly debilitating effect on a person's ability to think and feel in a way that is conducive to a productive, meaningful, and happy life.

The Connection to Anxiety and Depression

Tara's story provides a good example. Her pediatrician referred her for a sleep clinic evaluation because she had ongoing difficulty sleeping. Her sleep disturbances (multiple night awakenings, intermittent breathing difficulties, and snoring) had initially been interpreted by her parents as a form of anxiety. In fact, Tara was a normal child who was incorrectly labeled as anxious and depressed. She was sleep deprived when she was in school, and at the same time she was under physical pressure as her small body labored against the stenosis that was a result of her obesity. Her inadequate, fragmented sleep served as a stressor on her heart and on her family, who didn't understand this source of her mood changes.

Researchers believe that not getting enough sleep is likely to set the stage for negative thinking because the two main characteristics of depression, difficulty falling asleep and early morning awakening, cause a person to lose time in restorative sleep. Even some children with depression have abnormalities in their REM sleep. Experts explain that a lack of sleep often results in lower frustration thresholds and mood fluctuations. Children can be under further distress as they function in school and sometimes experience particularly negative reactions from parents or teachers who don't realize that this behavior may have a biological cause.

CHAPTER 7

Sleep and Physical Health

The correlation between too much sleep and general ill health is also very real. While the metabolic energy produced by the body for muscle movement clearly depends on fuel from not only sleep but food matters too, the concept doesn't completely account for all sleep/health connections. Experiments on sleep-deprived but well-fed laboratory animals demonstrate that their immune systems can't work properly after a time, which suddenly makes them vulnerable to frank illnesses, attacking the very energy suppliers—or at least the function of it—they need most. If one wanted to help the animals, the best thing to do would be to make sure they got their Zs, not push food at their faces.

Although scientists are only just beginning to connect the dots between insufficient sleep and deficits in physical health, the potential hazards of such connections are numerous and troubling indeed. At the most fundamental level, of course, there's the simple energy we need to get through the day. Energy powers everything done by the body and the brain. The food we eat provides fuel and the nutrients that enable us to convert that fuel into functional metabolic energy. Yet too little sleep may cause some of that fuel, in the form of glucose, to stay trapped in the bloodstream and never get to the muscle cells, which then desperately craves additional fuel to keep moving, keep powering the body within which they reside. Over time, such problems can build up and amplify to form the basis for type 2 diabetes and a potentially life-endangering family of heart problems, dubbed metabolic syndrome.

Immune Function

Cytokines are a crucial part of the immune system, playing the role of messengers conducting cell-to-cell communication. They help modulate an effective host response to pathogens. Sleep is essential for the normal regulation of the immune system and adequate quantity and quality sleep is crucial for the host defense mechanism. Research suggests that sleep has a multi-directional impact on the immune system: short sleep and poor quality sleep increase the risk of upper respiratory infections by affecting inflammation, production of cytokines, and lymphocytes (a type of white blood cell that helps produce antibodies to fight off infections). Longer sleeping times are associated with a decreased risk of upper respiratory symptoms. After exposure to both natural and experimental cold viruses, increased serum levels of proinflammatory cytokines such as IL-6 are associated with shorter sleep duration prior to viral challenge. Increased NREM sleep, in particular sleep spindles, were associated with increased next day feeling of being rested and reduced levels of specific proinflammatory cytokine (TNF-a). Inflammatory responses are beneficial in resolving infections and tissue damage but can also have negative effects, including fever, fatigue, and muscle pain. Forced waking before the natural waking may interfere with the immune system recovery and the associated benefits. Adequate sleep is necessary to enable the primary cytokine effect of repairing tissue damage to occur; sleep restriction may reduce the effectiveness of tissue repair. Sleep, therefore, can be seen as an anti-inflammatory effect.

Sleep has profound effects on your immune function. A lack of sleep is associated with the breakdown of the immune system. It has long been linked to an increase in susceptibility to illness, but more recently it has been demonstrated that sleep is essential to promote the beneficial inflammation that helps to repair the body from exposure to pathogens. That is not to say that more sleep is better in terms of immunity. More is not always better. Finding what is adequate to maximize your body's need can only be determined through experimentation. The relationship between sleep and immunity is complex and influenced by an athlete's training intensity and volume and nutrition. Although more research is needed to determine the optimal type of training, intensity, and volume and nutrition to support immunity, taking time to listen to your body's unique characteristics and know when it's time to back off, cross-train, or modify eating can help build a more resilient, healthy, and ultimately successful athlete.

CHAPTER 8

Sleep Hygiene and Best Practices

Good sleep hygiene can ensure that you maximize the benefits of sleep. This means more than just sleeping your six or eight hours. Good sleep quality and good sleep health also help to ensure that you awake refreshed, energized, and engaged in the new day to manage unexpected challenges as well as being ready to apply yourself to the process of concentration, learning, and recall. Good sleep hygiene can support both the restorative systems in the body related to sleep recharging health, as well as the metabolic systems related to less chronic illness. Being in management of your sleep health can lead to more success in those energy systems to help you build mental and emotional fortitude while at the same time promoting success in the process of biomedical learning. Have a stretch. Shake out the cobwebs. Stand tall with us and breathe in deeply. Let's make some commitments.

Welcome to the "Science of Sleep". We will share with you an understanding of what rest, sleep, and recharge do and do not do for the systems in the body, provide insight into human habits, lifestyle choices, and sleep disorders that may negatively impact our health. As healthcare professionals dedicated to helping to heal the body, mind, and spirit, we want every opportunity to provide important information that can help you to be as healthy as you can be. So rest with us, sleep on the thought-provoking, best healthy habits we will share, recharge, rejuvenate, and be ready to make choices that will help you thrive.

Creating a Sleep-Inducing Environment
While no studies have yet identified a given sound as particularly imperative for use in bedding that females will always give birth through labor by, say, the third lesson, bedroom sound seems likely to become another popular research area. However, our environment should no more awaken us spontaneously before this happy day than violate nature's ancient rhythms by dulling the cries of a newborn. First of all, choose silk fabrics. That dream state makes you sensually responsive; a silk comforter and pillowcase should nicely flatter your skin. Indeed, anything yielding or elastic is psychologically compatible with the cycle of sleep. A bouncy offer of defensibility and endurance damps noise while you sleep and guards peace if you wake up. In most situations, despite the intuitive appeal and full-market penetration of heavy, silencing draperies, a credible rating for serenity comes, courtesy of a wall-of-quiet.

Whether you sleep in a completely updated smart home or simply an old-fashioned bedroom, there are certain elements that any 21st-century bedroom should have in order to induce sleep. The key concerns are a setting that is conducive to all aspects of sleep hygiene: making the bedroom comfortable and supportive of their high-grand-guard goals about rest, sleep, and tranquility. To edge people toward emotional freedom and personal awakening is the central role of a therapeutic bedroom. The purpose is not only to encourage sleep and relaxation but to invite us into a different-consciousness climate. That being said, some high-tech toys might also be in order for some people. The trick with high technology is to use it in a way that enhances your sleep. Throughout history, including ancient Greece, enlightenment and peace were linked. Now scientific evidence exists that the tranquility of the personal environment and the tranquility of the psyche are linked too.

CHAPTER 9

Technology and Sleep

The 'Lights Off' Behind Excellent Sleep

At this stage, it is difficult to find someone who doesn't know how to operate a computer: press the power button or close the laptop to switch it off. It's locking it down that may be a different story for those with no one guiding them the first time. Why is it, then, that it is more difficult to understand that we, who are much older than any computer, should also turn off the lights? What is in light that interferes with sleep? The answer is that light, or better, a certain type of light - the short-wavelength or blue light - interferes with melatonin, the sleep hormone. Briefly, light controls the production of melatonin, made by the pineal gland in the brain.

The pineal gland 'listens' to the internal clock, a group of neurons that decides when is the right time to produce melatonin. The internal clock 'listens' to the light outside. In the light, the internal clock 'hears' that it is day's time and shuts melatonin off to let us feel awake. When it gets dark, or the color of the light becomes red, as it happens when the sun has set, the internal clock 'hears' that it is night, and 30 minutes after it got the message, melatonin begins to pop-up. Sunlight is rich in low-wavelength (or blue) light, and it is also the light emitted by most of the white-light-emitting diode (LED) backlit devices that fill our lives. Whether twitting on our smartphones, working on our computers, or watching the evening news, we are indeed enriched by the information we are exchanging, but our brains are not hearing about the coming of the dark night, and that's bad. The badness comes because with no melatonin, the neurons relax and fluff-up their sleep-provoking processing making rest difficult.

Blue Light and its Effects

The blue light produced by digital screens damages our circadian regulation. Young people are particularly sensitive to this. We don't yet understand the long-term effects of blue light on our health. Consequently, the issue at hand is colossal. We live in the information era and our digital screens are essential; they are our access points to knowledge, entertainment, and socialization. Yet it is clear, the use of backlit screens in the evening is a worrying activity. In particular, it disturbs the synthesis of melatonin, a hormone essential for our sleep. Researchers have studied this for years and have been able to define the factors which modulate blue light's ability to disturb our circadian rhythm.

Do you spend evenings staring at the artificial glow emanating from your computer screen? Then you are engaged in a risky activity which has far-reaching consequences on both your sleep and overall health. In a few years, we will have a formidable knowledge which will allow us to safely surf the internet in the total darkness of our bedrooms. Current research makes it clear: it is time to protect ourselves from the harmful effects of blue light once and for all.

CHAPTER 10

Sleep Across the Lifespan

Into adulthood, sleep and the development of sleep problems such as insomnia are influenced by a variety of factors including psychological stress and mood disorders, work schedules, and child-rearing demands. Many of these same factors interact with the aging process to influence sleep as we age. The role of sleep and the negative impacts of not getting enough sleep on memory and learning. Adolescence is a critical time for the consolidation of these cognitive functions and thus is a critical time for sleep. In addition to impairing memory and learning, lack of sleep during adolescence can lead to long-term consequences, including permanent changes in sleep and mood regulation that can carry through into adulthood. Small changes in school start time that allow for later wake-up calls and increased sleep lead to increased mood and memory in adolescents. The development of Alzheimer's disease is also influenced by sleep. Participants in the study who had self-reported shorter sleep duration and poorer sleep quality had increased buildup of toxins associated with Alzheimer's disease. We can begin to see the importance of sleep throughout our lives. It is not just a time to rest and recharge. It is a time to remember, to learn, to grow, to develop. These are important tasks. Would we deny them to our children or our elder generations?

Until this point, my focus has been on the adult and the circadian system, particularly with respect to the concepts of the homeostatic sleep drive and the window of opportunity for sleep each night. These are complex concepts, and there has been an explosion of research attempting to understand and manipulate important neurotransmitters involved in the sleep-wake cycle to promote sleep, both at the natural time and out of cap. But sleep is not only important for adults. Sleep is critical at all stages of life. Brain changes in infancy result in a fundamental difference in the sleep architecture of infants compared with older children and adults. As children grow into adolescence, there is a shift in sleep timing to prefer the nighttime hours, a result of changes in the circadian system and the sleep-wake system.

Sleep in Infants and Children
Newborns spend 16 to 18 hours per day sleeping. In 2-week-olds, this has increased to 14 to 18 hours, mainly because they are beginning to pace their activities into short bursts. 3-week-olds might sleep 15 hours per day but frequently awaken, while 6-week-old infants sleep 14 to 16 hours and wake up less often. By age 6 to 9 months, up to 1-year-olds typically sleep about 14 hours per day, with most of their sleep at night and increasing amounts of time without sleeping by day. By 3 years old, daytime napping is usually decreased from 3 to 1, and daytime napping is often eliminated by age 4.

The amount of sleep required changes as a person ages. There is a clear link between sleep and both mental and physical growth among infants and children. Different stages of sleep affect different aspects of growth, but sleep itself is required for infants to mature normally. Among children, sleep quality can have a direct impact on growth hormone levels, and by extension, growth. Sleep can also affect puberty in some cases, although researchers do not agree about how.

CHAPTER 11

Cultural and Societal Perspectives on Sleep

The interpretation of both the amount of sleep needed and the manner in which it is ritualistically obtained and maintained varies widely from one culture to another. Western societies seem most concerned with the number of hours of sleep per person, as indicated by an abundance of literature concerning the mysterious "average person." It is worth noting that experts believe that the average amount of sleep, whatever the correct value may be, is seriously underestimated. Both its restorative importance and the physical and psychosocial consequences of various degrees of sleep debt are frequently ignored as well.

Sleep, like many other facets of human existence, has a cultural component. In some societies, sleep is viewed as a passive, necessary act for the maintenance of physical health. Generally, controllers of all things professional regard sleep as incompatible with work, at least during the daytime. After a tough campaign or a long winter, political leaders often retreat for an extended period to rest and recuperate at a remote health spa or resort. In fact, it is not uncommon to hear people joke about politicians needing their rest. Conversely, in certain pioneering and emerging cultures where trying to sleep in a world of uncertainty and insecurity is not an option but a day-to-day challenge, sleep holds a completely different value and importance.

Sleep in Different Cultures

Shift worker bias, drugs, and lifestyle choices are radically affecting traditional sleeping times today. A Filipino factory worker may feel coerced by income essentials into sleeping away his natural lunchtime siesta, opting instead to snack on cigarettes in further ignorance about the unexpected detriments to his mental and physical health that are accumulating as a result. There appears to be no society on the planet that can't at least think about how to change so as to close the underappreciated gaps between the way their cultures currently sleep, and the way that they should sleep for optimum cognitive function and emotional health. As advocated by the science, every culture, particularly those in the authoritarian employment no-man's-land orthogonal to the daily solar rhythm, should openly debate these issues and affect sustainable change.

Different cultures have different attitudes toward sleep. Although Western cultures generally prize monophasic sleep, some 86 percent of the world's societies are actually polyphasic. These cultures encourage multiple naps embedded within their days, perhaps both to accommodate extreme heat and cold, and to help translate deeper, more sanctified sleep into a social bonding affair. Religious faith can also deeply influence a culture's relation with sleep. Jews, Muslims, Seventh-Day Adventists, and members of some Native American nations impose religious rituals on their sleep behavior, happily accepting the decreasing reliability of their brains to let them know when it is time to sleep as a natural threshold into their deity's responsibility. The Christian monastics, pre-Columbian Mexico's Otomi tribe, and several African cultures presented with the same problem praise the new lease on nocturnal life as a potential gateway to the sanctification of the following day.

CHAPTER 12

Sleep Research Methodologies

Currently, video- and infrared-based imaging are state-of-the-art methods applied in sleep studies for humans or for hand-scoring by sleep technologists. For animal or avian models, infrared thermography is used in sleep studies relegated to non-observable physiological parameters, while a video-based technique helps researchers exactly differentiate the stage of brain activity about animal slow-wave sleep or rapid eye movement sleep. The non-invasive advantage of brain imageries is beneficial for children, infants, or special clinical groups. To develop common knowledge, standardized feedback and real-time closed-loop research with integrated visualization and control interface are the critical next steps. Any available datasets or newly promulgated platforms may raise the significance of the future of integrated study. Interdisciplinary research will surely contribute to a definitive solution. Sleep-related issues, including insomnia, hypersomnia, and disturbances related to circadian rhythm, can then be suitably diagnosed through an optimized protocol. Technologies in the field of sleep monitoring and control systems can be extended into other horizons to mitigate a passenger's driving fatigue in the automotive industry, manage officer's working performance at the smart workplace, or intensify student focus and performance in the educational environment. In the healthcare area, early diagnosis, consistent treatment, and rapid recovery are also the themes for the next generation of sleep-enhanced tools.

Sleep research methodologies have evolved dramatically over the centuries, from observations and simple tools to state-of-the-art technologies. These revolutionary techniques have satisfied humanity's ongoing curiosity about the origins, functions, and mechanisms underlying sleep. Sleep researchers now employ the help of electrodes, computers, sophisticated recording devices, and the latest purpose-made hardware and software to measure, analyze, and interpret brain activity, electric impulses, movement, and biological rhythms throughout the night. In this chapter, sleep scoring, actigraphy techniques, and brain imaging methods shall be discussed. Various popular tools used in sleep research, ranging from behavioral assessments and polysomnographic analysis to brain stimulations, will be introduced. Emerging newly promising models, as well as challenges in the study of sleep states, yet remain open issues aggravated by other physiological and pathological conditions, will also be highlighted.

Polysomnography

The majority of patients presenting to sleep disorders clinics do so because of daytime sleepiness, disturbed nocturnal sleep, or due to snoring with or without a history of apneas noticed by the bed partner. The most common reason to perform polysomnography is the assessment of the impact of these sleep problems on the patient's ability to drive or the safety of his work or his peers. The use of clinical diagnosis based on a patient's history and complaints is notoriously unreliable in detecting the many sleep-related problems, and only by using multiple night PSG studies while addressing those confounding variables is it possible to obtain the quality of this often complex analysis mandated by a given patient's presenting complaints or concerns. The result of this analysis is the basis of patient treatment and management of sleep disorders. Establishing the ethical guidelines grounding sleep research can be found in Milliman and Qualitative EEG.

The most accurate work done on sleep disorders, particularly as these relate to organizational and pathophysiological issues, has been carried out using the measurement and associated analysis of the polysomnography sleep EEG. The term polysomnography denotes the study of sleep that monitors multiple channels including at least one electroencephalographic (EEG), electro-oculogram, and electromyographic recording. Sleep research, clinical or academic activities aimed at diagnosing or characterizing sleep pathologies on the basis of its effect on the patient's daily life should include extensive polysomnography sleep EEG (PSGn) studies.

CHAPTER 13

Future Trends in Sleep Science

One important consequence is that the drug companies must develop an understanding of the physiological mechanisms involved because otherwise they could inadvertently cause harmful side effects. So we will quickly learn more of sleep neurophysiology. As we understand more, we may tell all people to sleep longer. The traditional divide has been that insomnia is a disease that needs a cure, but that short sleep and sleep deprivation are simply consequences of being burned out. However, as we've seen, not sleeping enough is not good for you, contributing to obesity, diabetes, and perhaps even cardiovascular complications. There have not yet been good brain studies of overall sleep insufficiency, to find specifics of pathology and try to understand what sorts of people need more sleep than others and why.

As a science, sleep is still in its infancy. It was only in 1929 that it was discovered that we experienced four to six cycles of sleep in a night. There have been similar periods of discovery every 20-30 years. Brain waves were discovered in 1929, REM sleep was discovered in 1953, and the final piece to the puzzle, the REM sleep dreaming state, was discovered in 1959. Currently, we are still in a hot period of research on drugs to treat insomnia. At some point soon, we will probably declare victory, having a variety of different drugs and other treatments to meet the many needs different people have for controlling sleep. But drugs also help us more generally to understand the mechanisms of sleep. Melatonin caused a revolution in our understanding of circadian biology, so the development of drugs will probably help elucidate mechanisms of falling asleep and maintaining sleep more generally. Indeed, in the longer term, I suspect that the main use of drugs will be to help understand more about mechanisms and about the implications of deficient sleep.

Emerging Technologies

Other consumer products that monitor some aspect of sleep physiology include the Sleeptracker wristwatch, and the Humana-Dossier bed sensor. Another consumer-friendly EEG monitor now available is from a company called Emotiv, whose headset is used primarily as a neuro-feedback controller in research, gaming, and artistic applications. Keep in mind that collecting sleep data is only a first step for all of these devices and apps. What really matters is what you do with that data, and the potential for these devices goes much further than simply data collection. The WakeMate has a built-in smart alarm to gently wake you when you're in a lighter stage of sleep, the Arousal Promoting Feedback system uses the under-the-pillow sensor to trigger mild vibrations when the system detects that the sleeper is snoring, which is usually a signal of disordered breathing or other sleep disturbance.

The devices and apps we listed merely scratch the surface of the burgeoning world of sleep-related technologies. Also on the market today is a small headband from Zeo, a company co-founded by several sleep researchers. The device has that same familiar sensor that rests on the forehead to pick up brain wave information while the slowly oscillating colored orb sitting next to your bed acts as a reminder to you that you're not asleep every time you change position (no doubt, this is a comforting thing to watch). Grabbing this information allows the device to report on how much slow wave and REM sleep you've managed to grab that night while you slept. Like the WakeMate, the company offers a software solution, turning monitoring data to help track potential sleep issues and optimize your own sleep environment. This bi-directional feedback is the exciting part of both of these devices, and we envision a time when there will be an open API that combines the systems and data these devices generate to offer ever-more-powerful ways to really dig deeper into these health-supporting systems.

CHAPTER 14

Conclusion and Practical Tips for Better Sleep

I am a big advocate of medicine: the benefits far outweigh the costs. But I am also a die-hard believer in the intellectuals of the brain, in its power of self-repair if we just give it some time and respect. For instance, 99 percent of people with insomnia show major improvement in their emotion-regulating skills and sleep quality when going through cognitive behavioral therapy for insomnia (CBT-I). Such a non-pharmacological treatment involves teaching insomniacs how to get out of their wings of thinking when faced with rumination about sleep, thus facilitating their learning of more realistic and adaptive beliefs about sleep patterns. These are learned skills that should last a lifetime. Why are we not seeing these clinical programs become more widespread, resulting in a similar chaos about insomnia treatment efficacy as we currently see about nutrition? I don't have an answer, unfortunately. But I do propose that it's time to rebuild the case for a renaissance of sleep education as a science priority.

Sleep is sometimes referred to as a "soft science," but in truth, the recent advances in our understanding of sleep, both at the brain level and at the clinical and psychiatric levels, have made it into a very hard science. These are not your grandmother's "over my eyes" findings about sleep. The unfolding story involves constant revision of the old belief systems about sleep, showing that it is not a simple process, nor does it exist in a theoretical silence void of our other major life domains. A comprehensive understanding of sleep requires connections to be made between body, mind, and soul. It doesn't help to complain about being tired all the time or to be embarrassed about it. And it definitely does not help in the long run to think that anti-anxiety or anti-depressant medications are suitable long-term solutions for sleep problems.

www.ingramcontent.com/pod-product-compliance
Lightning Source LLC
LaVergne TN
LVHW092100060526
838201LV00047B/1479